Succeeding in Academic Medicine Applications

Succeeding in Academic Medicine Applications

Rele Ologunde

Academic Clinical Fellow in Otolaryngology,
University Hospitals Birmingham NHS Foundation
Trust and University of Birmingham

Scion

© Scion Publishing Limited, 2019

ISBN 9781911510345

First published 2019

A CIP catalogue record for this book is available from the British Library.

Scion Publishing Limited

The Old Hayloft, Vantage Business Park, Bloxham Road, Banbury OX16 9UX, UK

www.scionpublishing.com

Important Note from the Publisher

The information contained within this book was obtained by Scion Publishing Ltd from sources believed by us to be reliable. However, while every effort has been made to ensure its accuracy, no responsibility for loss or injury whatsoever occasioned to any person acting or refraining from action as a result of information contained herein can be accepted by the authors or publishers.

Although every effort has been made to ensure that all owners of copyright material have been acknowledged in this publication, we would be pleased to acknowledge in subsequent reprints or editions any omissions brought to our attention.

Registered names, trademarks, etc. used in this book, even when not marked as such, are not to be considered unprotected by law.

Cover design by Andrew Magee Design Ltd
Typeset by Evolution Design & Digital Ltd (Kent)
Printed in the UK

Last digit is the print number: 10 9 8 7 6 5 4 3 2 1

CONTENTS

PREFACE

Success doesn't come from being a hundred percent better than your competition, but from being one percent better in a hundred different ways.

– ANON –

A career in academic medicine is in equal parts rewarding and challenging. The opportunity to be involved in driving through research that underpins our understanding of complex diseases and trialling novel therapeutic interventions is thrilling yet demanding. However, as a clinical academic the pursuit of research interests cannot be done at the expense of attaining excellence in clinical competencies. As such, the demands of an academic career put many off. However, those who choose this path no doubt share a common longing and fulfilment from pursuing uncharted waters. This journey involves constantly learning, all with the end goal of advancing our understanding of disease and illness, bettering medical practice and improving patient outcomes. Ultimately the adventure into the unknown comes with the greatest risk but also the greatest potential and sense of fulfilment.

The National Institute of Health Research (NIHR) integrated academic training pathway formalised academic training in the UK in 2006 with the creation of a run-through training pathway that incorporated both clinical and academic competencies. The integrated pathway is a unique opportunity to create alignment between academics and clinicians, bringing direct patient relevance to translational scientific research. Recruitment to all stages of this pathway is extremely competitive and as such, academic positions attract a great deal of prestige. Successful candidates will often go on to have long-lasting and fruitful careers in academia. However, enjoyment of such a career does not have to be limited to a privileged few.

If you are reading this book you are no doubt motivated to give yourself the greatest possible chance of securing your dream academic job and excelling in it. Succeeding at interview and during your academic programme is about preparing and practising the right way. Too many good candidates fail to demonstrate just how good they really are and therefore miss out. However, preparing to succeed doesn't begin once you get an interview or even when you begin to consider applying for an academic post. Preparing to succeed starts much earlier on. To this end, the first half of this book focuses on the things that you can do to put yourself in the best position possible, years before that interview. The second half of the book discusses the ways in which to excel at interview and in your academic career. Anecdotally, many consultants who participate in national selection for trainee posts often comment that they can tell whether a person will be successful or not, simply based on the level and quality of evidence within their portfolio. For candidates not performing as strongly on other aspects of the selection process, the portfolio provides a strong boost to the overall score. As such, a significant portion of this book is devoted to ways in which your portfolio can be improved to set you apart from others and dramatically improve your chances of success.

This book has been put together using insights from successful trainees, to allow all applicants to benefit from advice that comes only from experience; it focuses on teaching the skills that produce results rather than the knowledge.

Good luck in your future academic career!

Rele Ologunde

ACKNOWLEDGEMENTS

Writing this book was harder than I thought but more rewarding than I could have imagined. I am eternally grateful to my parents for their constant support, sacrifice and prayers; my wife, Vicky, for her patience and forbearance and my brother for his guidance and wisdom.

I would like to thank James Glasbey for his insight and thoughts that helped shape this book. Lastly, I would like to thank Dr Jonathan Ray and Clare Boomer at Scion Publishing, without whom this book would not have been possible.

ABBREVIATIONS

ACF	Academic Clinical Fellowship
AFP	Academic Foundation Programme
AUoA	Academic Unit of Application
CL	Clinical Lectureship
CPD	Continuing Professional Development
FP	Foundation Programme
FY	Foundation year
GCP	good clinical practice
GMC	General Medical Council
IATP	Integrated Academic Training Pathway
M&M	morbidity and mortality
MRes	Masters in Research
NIHR	National Institute for Health Research
PROM	Patient Reported Outcome Measure
QoL	quality of life
RCT	randomised controlled trial
ST	Specialty Trainee
STARSurg	Student Audit and Research in Surgery
UKFPO	United Kingdom Foundation Programme Office
WBA	workplace-based assessment

CHAPTER 1

Introduction to academic medicine

If the pathway to success were well lit
it would already be crowded.

– ANON –

The evolution and advancement of medicine over the ages is underpinned by the curiosity and drive of those daring individuals who were never satisfied to accept the boundaries of their knowledge. Individuals who push on to find answers to the questions that people have not even begun to ask. Medicine is a unique vocation whereby research and clinical practice inform one another on a constant basis and drive change in a synergistic and reciprocal fashion. As such, it is a necessity that all medical professionals have an appreciation and understanding of the role and process of research in improving patient care and outcomes. Research has therefore begun to take a position of greater prominence in the training of medical professionals, with more opportunities for training in research governance, methodologies and collaborative work amongst trainees.

Clinicians pursuing academic careers play a crucial role in broadening our understanding of disease and health. Maintaining the health of local populations rests, in part, on the contributions that clinical academics make to scholarly activities such as research and clinical education. However, recruitment of junior trainees into academic careers within medicine remains a concern. In 1973, a decline in interest in academia amongst UK medical students was first highlighted, and this decline continues to be observed in other countries. As of 2013, only 6% of the UK medical workforce were recognised as clinical academics.

Historically, doctors choosing to pursue an academic career had to forge their own 'novel' career pathways, with no provision in place for balancing the competing requirements for training in both academia and clinical research. Often these doctors were scrutinised against the achievements of their full-time colleagues in academia and medicine, despite having effectively half the time to achieve comparable outputs. As such, a long-standing challenge of pursuing a career in academic medicine has been the lack of a formal training pathway. To this end it was apparent that academic medicine needed a revival. The Savill and Walport Reports were commissioned to investigate the demise of academic medicine and duly highlighted the need to increase the recruitment and training of academic clinicians in the UK. These reports culminated in the creation of the National Institute for Health Research (NIHR) in 2006, and of the Scottish Clinical Research Excellence Development Scheme in 2009. The NIHR set out to formalise training in academic medicine and established the UK Academic Foundation Programme (AFP). The AFP was designed to be a two-year postgraduate clinical training programme for newly qualified doctors. This would provide protected time to explore a career in academic medicine through the development of skills in research, management / leadership, or education. The AFP was piloted in 2005. Academic foundation year 2 (FY2) jobs were fully introduced in August 2006 and joined by academic foundation year 1 (FY1) jobs and Academic Clinical Fellowships (ACF) in August 2007.

The combination of academic training gained alongside clinical training, with protected time in which to pursue the academic activities, thus provided a formal training pathway for clinical academics known as the NIHR Integrated Academic Training Pathway (IATP) for doctors and dentists (*Figure 1.1*). The AFP thus serves as a possible entry point to the IATP. This training pathway is extremely flexible, allowing trainees to enter and exit at various points in the pathway and stages in their career, should they need to do so.

Successful completion of an AFP, non-academic foundation programme or recognised equivalent enables candidates to apply for an ACF and formally enter the IATP.

- ACFs typically last three years (four years for General Practice), with the aim of preparing trainees for application for a higher degree such as a PhD, DPhil or MD.
- Upon completion of the higher degree, or for trainees already holding such a degree, the next stage of the training pathway is a Clinical Lectureship (CL), which lasts four years.

Currently, ACF trainees spend 75% of their time in clinical training, with the rest being in academia. CL trainees typically spend equal amounts of time in clinical and academic practice. As of 2018, there are approximately 500 AFPs, 250 ACFs and 80 CLs advertised each year.

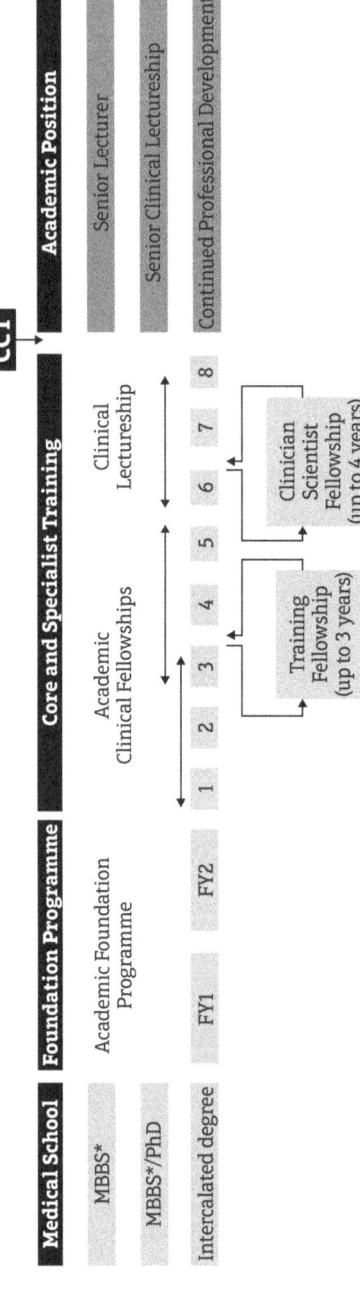

CCT: Certificate of Completion of Training
Personal fellowships can be undertaken at any point during training.
* or equivalent medical degree (e.g. MBChB)

Figure 1.1 Integrated Academic Training Pathway (IATP). Reproduced with permission from Ologunde, R., Sismey, G. and Kelley, T. (2018) The UK Academic Foundation Programmes: are the objectives being met? *Journal of the Royal College of Physicians of Edinburgh*, 48(1): 54–61.

1.1   Why undertake academic training?

A career as a clinician–academic isn't for everyone, but research experience is certainly beneficial throughout all stages of your career. The ability to develop skills in the critical appraisal of evidence will be of benefit when informing your own clinical practice, or when describing the relative merits of various types of treatment to your patient. Research experience also provides the opportunity to further develop understanding and expertise in a specialist area which, in addition to being rewarding, can also demonstrate your commitment to that particular area or sub-specialism. A commitment to research will also help to drive up standards locally, by implementing evidence-based medicine for the benefit of patients. Furthermore, improvements in standards may even be seen regionally or perhaps further afield.

The transferable skills that clinical academics undertaking research accrue over time are considerable, although perhaps difficult to quantify. These include skills in statistical analysis, time management, public speaking and presentation, project implementation, and the commitment and dedication that come with taking a research question from inception to completion. Some even get to publish the results of multi-centre, international randomised controlled trials (RCTs) in a major journal.

Research encompasses more than just laboratory-based experiments, although this is what frequently comes to mind when undergraduates are asked about their impression of research. However, it extends right through to clinical work, even including patients at the design stage of studies before recruitment begins. Research also includes qualitative aspects, epidemiological trends and theoretical concepts, such as those underpinning medical education pedagogy.

1.2 A day in the life of an academic

Days of work as a clinical academic can be extremely variable and will very much depend at what stage in your training you are and what type of research you are involved in. As such, a typical day seldom exists in reality, but to give you an idea of what you might expect as an AFP doctor or as an ACF, a couple of examples are shown in *Boxes 1.1* and *1.2*.

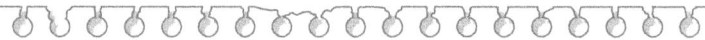

Box 1.1 A day in the life of an AFP doctor

Dr John Lee Allen, undertaking clinical research in otolaryngology in Oxford.

07:00 – breakfast and make a plan for the week ahead.
My academic time took the form of a 'day release', often on a Monday, so there was plenty to plan and fit in during that day before returning to clinical duties.

08:00 – work on abstract / funding grant applications.
I would make careful note of any deadlines and use free time during the day to meet with collaborators.

09:00 – discuss ideas and progress with academic supervisor.
I would usually make a target for what I would want to complete by the following week.

10:00 – review literature and work on data analysis for a global surgical safety research project.
This involved learning how to use the statistical program R to automatically generate reports for hospitals that were members of the collaborative team.

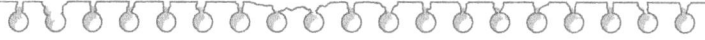

12:00 – give a presentation at group lunchtime research meeting and get useful feedback on analysis/future research directions.

13:00 – meet with clinical supervisor to discuss Quality Improvement Project ideas.
This is part of the foundation training portfolio and it was useful to be able to meet during the day whilst not engaged with clinical duties.

14:00 – medical school clinical skills teaching.
This was a convenient way to engage with the university teaching programme because it was conducted on the hospital site.

15:00 – continue work on data analysis and meet with colleagues working on similar analyses.

18:00 – dinner in college with academic colleagues to discuss progress and other academic opportunities.
This was a useful source of information for clinical and academic portfolio building.

19:00 – mock examinations teaching in college.
This was a great way to be part of the college teaching programme and to see a cohort of students through their clinical examinations.

21:00 – attend weekly video conference call with global research collaborative to discuss the database and preparation for the annual conference.

22:00 – prepare for the next day of clinical work.

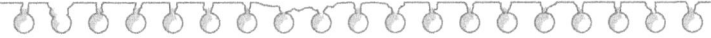

Box 1.2 A day in the life of an academic clinical fellow

Mr James Glasbey, undertaking clinical trials in colorectal and global surgery research in Birmingham.

05:45 – wake up, quick shower.

06:15 – breakfast, strong coffee and a catch up with eTable of Contents notifications from my favourite journals.

07:00 – walk to work, catch up with collaborative research group WhatsApp threads and respond to any project queries.

07:30 – review my diary for the day and plan my 'Next Actions'.

07:45 – early morning meeting with our Professor of Surgery to discuss progress with an analysis from our completed RCT in colorectal cancer.

08:30 – spend the morning performing analysis of our latest international cohort study of post-operative surgical outcomes using the R Studio statistics program and preparing a manuscript for peer-reviewed publication.

11:30 – International Trial Management Group meeting for our ongoing international trial in reduction of surgical wound infection; joined by 30 surgeons from 22 low- and middle-income countries. Planning for site set-up and troubleshooting trial delivery.

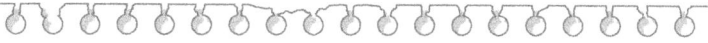

13:30 – lunch with colleagues from my surgical research team. More strong coffee!

14:00 – meet my intercalated BSc student to plan her research project for the coming year, and guide her application for competitive grant funding.

14:30 – Masters in Research (MRes) module seminar on Project Management and Research Governance (funding is included within the ACF post award).

16:00 – visit the Birmingham Clinical Trials Unit to meet with multidisciplinary colleagues in research methodology (health economists, trial methodologists and statisticians) to discuss protocol design for a new NIHR-funded trial.

18:00 – rush home in time for a CrossFit workout.

19:30 – teleconference and troubleshooting with regional leads of our latest medical student-led collaborative research study.

20:00 – relax at home and cook dinner with my girlfriend.

Further reading

- The Academy of Medical Sciences (2000) *The Tenured Track Clinician Scientist: a new career pathway to promote recruitment into academic medicine* (the **Savill Report**). London: AMS.
- Lawson McLean, A., Saunders, C., Velu, P.P. *et al.* (2013) Twelve tips for teachers to encourage student engagement in academic medicine. *Medical Teacher*, **35(7):** 549–54.
- Modernising Medical Careers and the UK Clinical Research Collaboration (2005) *Medically- and Dentally-qualified Academic Staff: recommendations for training the researchers and educators of the future.* Report of the Academic Careers Sub-committee of Modernising Medical Careers and the UK Clinical Research Collaboration (the **Walport Report**). Available at: www.ukcrc.org/wp-content/uploads/2014/03/Medically_and_Dentally-qualified_Academic_Staff_Report.pdf
- NIHR (2017) *Guide to National Institute for Health Research Integrated Academic Training* v.1.1 ('NIHR Gold Guide'). Available at: www.nihr.ac.uk/funding-and-support/documents/IAT/TCC-NIHR-IAT-GUIDE.pdf

CHAPTER 2

Maximising the medical school years

By failing to prepare, you are preparing to fail.

– BENJAMIN FRANKLIN –

It is never too late to decide to pursue an academic career and there are merits and disadvantages whenever you decide to start. For those of you reading this book whilst still at medical school – you have the benefit of time, and only in hindsight will you realise this. However, there are disadvantages and challenges to committing to a niche field of research early on in your career, such as reduced clinical knowledge to inform your choice of research field and the possibility of prolonging your training, should you choose to intercalate or do a higher degree.

Pre-clinical medical training is an ideal time to begin considering pursuing an academic career. Despite the seemingly endless lists of diseases, processes and eponymous syndromes that you have to learn, there is relatively more time for the pursuit of extracurricular activity compared to later on in your career. In this chapter we will briefly explore how you can get involved in research as a student. We will explore further the specifics of maximising academic opportunities in *Chapter 4*.

2.1 Conferences

Approaching a research supervisor is often a daunting prospect but there are ways in which you can make this much easier. One way of doing this during pre-clinical training is by joining specialty and sub-specialty organisations and attending their relevant meetings. These meetings give you not only the opportunity to network with other colleagues and esteemed individuals in your field of interest, but also the opportunity to hear about the latest research developments in these fields and ideas with which to develop your own research questions and hypotheses to test.

These conferences also provide an opportunity for you to present your own research projects and will typically only require the submission of a short abstract, often less than 500 words. When it comes to interview, as we will see later on in this book, presentations at national and international conferences carry a significant amount of weight and are looked upon extremely favourably during the interview selection process. Many conferences also offer heavily subsidised rates for students and it is often far cheaper to attend the conference several times as a student, and equally, present on multiple occasions, than to attend even once as a qualified doctor.

2.2 Courses

Increasingly, extra-curricular courses are being run by specialty and private organisations. These courses vary from being specialty-focused, such as those teaching surgical skills and instrument handling, to courses focusing on teaching skills. A number of courses offer discounted rates for students, and some are even free. Many courses are advertised by Royal Colleges and societies and other national bodies on their websites. It is very worthwhile joining the relevant mailing lists of these organisations in order to keep abreast of the courses on offer.

If you have a particularly niche area of interest and are unable to find a course on the subject matter, consider setting up a course yourself. Most universities allow students and student societies to hire rooms on campus free or for a nominal fee. You can then invite an expert in the field to deliver a talk or workshop. This serves to address the deficit in terms of meeting an intellectual need for the course, and you can list course organisation as an item of evidence in your portfolio; this will be discussed further in *Chapter 4*.

2.3   Research projects

Many universities offer undergraduate research opportunity programmes that run during the summer vacation. These typically vary from four to eight weeks and often attract a stipend to cover research and subsistence costs. The Academy of Medical Sciences, through their INSPIRE scheme, also provides dedicated funding to all UK medical schools specifically to support the delivery of activities and programmes aimed at promoting a potential career in research. Increasingly, medical and surgical specialty organisations and Royal Colleges advertise research studentships which typically constitute a bursary to support research activities within the UK and overseas. These opportunities are typically open to medical students at all stages of training.

Furthermore, with the creation of the Student Audit and Research in Surgery (STARSurg) there have never been more collaborative opportunities to engage in research as a student. STARSurg is a student-led audit and research network active throughout the UK and Ireland. With an ever-increasing research portfolio and regular academic and research training, the STARSurg model helps to promote evidence-based practice in early training, which will hopefully inspire and enthuse potential future academics.

2.4 Prizes

Prizes provide a great way to add significant achievement to your CV, and some prizes can be won with relatively little effort on your part. A number of national medical organisations, colleges and associations run annual prizes specifically aimed at medical students. For example, the Royal Society of Medicine offers numerous annual prizes, some of which require only the submission of a research abstract. For those who may find good quality research projects difficult to come by, essay prizes are a great way to build on your academic CV. Some essay prizes also offer publication of the winning essay in a peer-reviewed journal, so one essay could potentially get you both a token prize and a publication.

2.5 Added value activities

In addition to those highlighted in *Sections 2.2* to *2.4*, there are a number of unique opportunities for bolstering your academic CV during your medical school years. During academic interviews and indeed most interviews where you will be taking on a more senior role, you will be asked for evidence of leadership. To this end, it is vital to begin to amass the evidence as early as possible. Whilst at medical school the ways in which you may show your leadership skills include being actively involved in university student societies or sitting on regional or national committees as a student representative. Furthermore, you may decide to lead or organise events or courses for your peers, or consider taking a lead role in extra-curricular activities such as advocacy or, for example, promoting medicine, first aid or CPR training in schools.

Further reading

- Academy of Medical Sciences, INSPIRE scheme – https://acmedsci.ac.uk/grants-and-schemes/mentoring-and-other-schemes/INSPIRE
- Royal Society of Medicine prizes and awards – www.rsm.ac.uk/prizes-and-awards
- Student Audit and Research in Surgery (STARSurg) collaborative – https://starsurg.org

CHAPTER 3

The application process (AFP and ACF)

Choice, not chance, determines your destiny.

− ARISTOTLE −

In the UK, application to the Academic Foundation Programme and Academic Clinical Fellowships are coordinated through Oriel, an online portal for recruitment to postgraduate medical, dental, public health, healthcare science and pharmacy training programmes. The portal allows you to view vacancies, complete application forms, book interviews and accept offers of appointment.

3.1 Academic Foundation Programme (AFP)

Applicants for the Academic Foundation Programme are currently nominated by their medical school as being eligible to apply, and in the main, this eligibility extends to all candidates who have completed the course successfully up to the point of application. Applicants holding, or due to be awarded, a primary medical degree from a non-UK university need to apply for assessment of eligibility directly to the United Kingdom Foundation

Programme Office (UKFPO). Applicants are then invited to register and apply for the Academic Foundation Programme, typically in the autumn of each year.

Applications to the AFP typically open earlier than applications to the (non-academic) foundation programme, and candidates can apply for both. At the time of writing, applicants are asked to register for an Oriel account and choose two (out of fifteen) Academic Units of Application (AUoAs). AUoAs broadly represent partnerships between foundation schools and their affiliated universities and are divided geographically across the UK. The application form varies depending on the AUoA that you are applying to and their particular areas of interest and enquiry.

Choosing an Academic Unit of Application

It is important to do your research on the AFP that each AUoA offers as they do differ, both in terms of research focus and of how academic time is protected and delivered. Some AUoAs allow applicants to devise their own research topic, whereas others may have set projects for applicants to take up. Both have merit but it is important not to commit yourself to two years of academic training on a project in which you have little interest. Conversely, if you do not have a particular desire to pursue a specific field of research or develop a project that you have previously worked on, a ready-made project may suit you. You may also find it useful to speak to previous academic trainees who have completed the programme in the area to which you wish to apply.

Academic achievements

The application form for the AFP allows candidates to provide evidence of additional academic achievement. The specifics may vary from one AUoA to another, but by and large most will allow you to provide evidence for the following categories:

- Higher postgraduate degrees attained (e.g. MSc, MD, PhD)
- Presentation of a poster at a regional, national or international meeting
- Giving an oral presentation at a regional, national or international meeting
- Prizes for academic excellence within medical school
- National or international prizes
- Outstanding achievement in an extra-curricular activity
- Research or travel fellowships (excluding elective bursaries or prizes).

In scoring candidates' additional academic achievements, AUoAs will vary in how much credit they give each item of evidence. The academic prospectus of each AUoA may provide further guidance in this regard.

'White space' questions

White space questions are so called because they are open-ended, requiring a free text response. As such, they are considered a more challenging part of the AFP application with no clear 'correct' answer. In truth, there are no wrong answers but certainly some answers are better than others. The advantage of this part of the application is that it gives you an opportunity to make your application stand out from others, beyond the number of academic accolades accrued. However, not all AUoAs include white space questions.

Typically, the questions asked in this section vary between AUoAs and are only available to view and respond to for a time-limited period during the application process. During this time, you can save your answers and return to the application.

Questions asked by AUoAs in the 'white space' section tend to focus on similar themes, including – but not limited to – research, teaching, management, motivations for the AFP, teamwork and contribution to academia during medical school.

Example 'white space' questions:

- Describe your research experience to date.
- Describe your teaching and/or management experience to date.
- Give an example of a research project, management or teaching experience and its significance to your application for the AFP.
- What are the teaching and research skills that you would most like to take away from your AFP? Outline your strategy for acquiring or developing these skills.
- Describe a time, that will be relevant to your foundation training, when you have worked as a successful member of a team and identify your role and contribution to this success.
- Give an example to describe your contribution to academic life during your medical school career and how it will be relevant to an academic medical career.
- Describe your academic and non-academic achievements and their significance to your application.
- Describe how you would set out to answer a research question that has arisen from a specific clinical case that you have been involved in.
- How would training on the AFP contribute to your overall career goals?

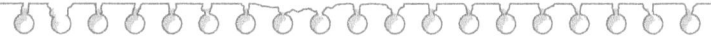

Box 3.1 Example of an excellent answer to a white space question

QUESTION: What are the teaching and research skills (maximum of three) that you would most like to take away from this Academic Programme, and that you do not already have? Briefly outline your strategy for acquiring or developing these skills.

ANSWER: I would like to develop my understanding of educational theory by undertaking a formal qualification in education such as a Postgraduate Diploma in Higher Education, as offered by the University Learning Institute. I would also like to consolidate this by further developing my teaching skills through the medical school Teacher Development Programme.

To date I have had relatively little formal teaching in statistics and so I would be keen to access the medical statistics course through the Academic Foundation Programme (AFP). Having spoken to previous AFP doctors in the region, I understand that there are a wealth of courses available to local trainees, and I would seek to register for these early on so that I can gain skills to complement my research activities.

I would also like to improve my skills in epidemiology. I would go about doing this by enrolling on relevant courses offered by the university. I would then put these skills into practice by undertaking a research project consisting of analysis of epidemiological data, in line with my interests in craniofacial surgery. I would, for example, complete an evaluation of the causes and incidence of maxillofacial injuries in the UK in the last ten years.

The answer given to the question in *Box 3.1* is good, for a number of reasons. Firstly, the question clearly asks for a maximum of three teaching and research skills and the candidate has listed and expanded on exactly three. Clearly there are no additional marks to be gained from listing any more than the number specifically asked for. Secondly, the candidate has chosen a mix of both teaching and research skills, thereby addressing both aspects of the question. Lastly, and perhaps most importantly, the candidate has outlined a clear strategy for how they would acquire these skills. Furthermore, they have given specific examples of how they would then put these newly acquired skills to use during their academic programme. The candidate has successfully and succinctly addressed all aspects of the questions asked, with specific examples given where appropriate.

Box 3.2 Example of a poor answer to a white space question

QUESTION: Academic medicine requires an individual to work successfully in a team. Describe a time, relevant to your foundation training, when you worked as a successful member of a team and identify your role and contribution to this success.

ANSWER: As a core committee member of my medical school Surgical Society I participated in the running of our national surgical conference. I had been delegated a specific role to oversee the running of a practical station in basic surgical skills (BSS). I had to liaise with other committee members to ensure that the timings of the workshop did not overrun onto the allocated time of workshops occurring simultaneously. This allowed my colleagues, who were coordinating the concurrent workshops, to confidently plan the timings of their own stations. I also developed a successful working relationship with the surgical trainees facilitating the BSS workshop. I ensured that equipment was prepared well in advance of delegates arriving, whilst also regularly replenishing consumables. My time management skills and proactive approach to resourcing equipment ensured that the workshop ran to time and was well equipped. My experience of working in multiple teams simultaneously during the conference has greatly improved my interpersonal, conflict resolution and priority setting skills. These skills will help me in being able to successfully oversee tasks that have been delegated to me whilst liaising with numerous members of a clinical team.

Although the answer given above describes how the candidate has worked in a team and the skills that they have gained from the experience, the answer suffers from one of the basic cardinal errors that individuals often make in applications; they have failed to actually answer the question. Firstly, the question asks for a description of a time that would be relevant to foundation training. Whilst you may well arrange teaching courses and other extra-curricular activities during foundation training, this is beyond the scope and focus of foundation training. As such, the example given by the candidate lacks relevance to the question being asked.

It is useful to draft answers to 'white space' questions early and ask colleagues or friends, both medical and non-medical, to read them for clarity and understanding. As a rule of thumb, a good approach to seeking feedback on your work is to adopt a 'pyramid of feedback' approach, whereby you start at the bottom and work your way up. You would thereby initially seek peer feedback, then near peer feedback, then input from a senior academic or clinical colleague and finally, if possible, perhaps from a more established colleague, such as a consultant or professor. At each stage of the pyramid you would revise your draft in light of the comments received. There are numerous frameworks that may help with formulating answers to questions such as those described above and a good reference text for this is *Medical Interviews* by Olivier Picard *et al.*, details of which are given in the further reading section at the end of this chapter.

Once the window for submission of applications has closed, AUoA will shortlist candidates based on predefined criteria. Applicants will receive one of the following outcomes: offer of an interview, being put on the waiting list, or application unsuccessful.

Successful AFP applicants will receive offers from AUoAs in advance of the Foundation Programme (FP) allocation process, and those who accept their offer will not be included in the FP allocation. Unsuccessful AFP applicants, or those who decline all AFP offers, will be included automatically in the FP allocation. If an applicant accepts an AFP offer and then decides to decline it, the applicant will be withdrawn from the entire process, including FP.

3.2   Academic Clinical Fellowship (ACF)

The application process of the Academic Clinical Fellowship is much the same as that of the AFP, discussed in *Section 3.1*. ACFs are offered in a number of specialties and start at differing times during training, most commonly at ST1 (Specialty Trainee year 1, following foundation training) and ST3 (after core training in medicine or surgery). All ACFs are advertised on Oriel and applications typically open in the autumn of each year.

Choosing an ACF

Academic Clinical Fellowships vary greatly, both in the focus of the research project (clinical vs. laboratory) and also in the way academic time is split. Furthermore, some ACFs come with the expectation that successful applicants will undertake a higher degree, such as an MSc or MRes, alongside their ACF. In most cases funding will be provided as part of the ACF to cover the costs of the higher degree.

It is also important to choose a geographical location that is compatible with your long-term goals. Unlike AFPs, which only last two years, an ACF is a six- to eight-year commitment, depending on what stage of training you start the programme. Upon completion of the three-year ACF you will return to full-time clinical training unless you defer, to take time out for a PhD or other activity.

Finally, it is also useful to do some research about the supervisor of the ACF and the research team that you will be working in. It may even be worthwhile arranging an informal meeting to find out more about the programme and work of the research team.

Academic application

Once you have shortlisted the ACFs you wish to apply to, you will have to complete an application for each individually. Some of the content in the applications may overlap. You will typically be asked to provide three referees: a Consultant or Educational Supervisor from your current employment, someone to provide you with an academic reference, and another referee from your medical training. You will then be asked to provide an employment history going back to the date of your primary medical qualification.

Academic achievements

As with the application for the AFP, candidates applying for the ACF are asked to list additional academic achievements. However, ACF applications tend to be more prescriptive about what they require. The following categories are examples of additional academic achievements that may be included in an ACF application:

- Additional completed undergraduate and postgraduate degrees and qualifications
- Undergraduate and postgraduate prizes, awards and distinctions
- Training courses relevant to your specialty of application that you have attended, and details of courses that you are currently undertaking
- Outstanding achievements outside the field of medicine
- Relevant presentations in your specialty of application
- Relevant publications in your specialty of application.

Most applications will ask you to state whether the presentations that you list in your application were poster or oral presentations and whether they were delivered to a local body or a regional or national society. Similarly, with publications most applications will ask for full citation details, including a PubMed link or alternative. For both presentations and publications, many applications will also ask you to state your role in or contribution to the work (e.g. first author, primary investigator).

'White space' questions

As with the AFP application, ACF applications have a varying number of white space questions. These cover similar themes to those in the AFP application, such as research, teaching, management and motivations for the ACF.

Example 'white space' questions:

- What experience do you have of delivering teaching? This may include a teaching skills course or a formal qualification in teaching, if undertaken.
- What is your experience of clinical audit to date?
- Describe how you believe you meet the person specification

for the programme you are applying for. Include the particular skills and attributes that make you suitable for a career in this specialty.

- Provide evidence of activities and achievements which demonstrate your commitment to a career in this specialty and/or have led to the development of skills relevant to a career in this specialty.
- Give brief details of all research projects and/or relevant research experience that you have undertaken or are undertaking, including methods used. Indicate your level of involvement and your exact role in the research team, detailing when this took place, your time commitment, your contribution / involvement and source of funding.
- Describe why you want this particular Academic Clinical Fellowship, indicating your medium- and long-term career goals in relation to an academic career in this specialty area.

Shortlisting

The shortlisting panel for each ACF will vary in how much credit or emphasis they place on different aspects of the application form, when it comes to determining candidates to invite for interview. The additional documents provided on Oriel for each application may provide further guidance. Once shortlisting has been completed, applicants are either offered an interview, put on the waiting list or are unsuccessful.

It is worthwhile reading through the NIHR Academic Clinical Fellowship Guidance for Recruitment and Appointment, which is updated annually, for the most recent person specification, interview scoring criteria, and essential and desirable applicant criteria. This guide is available to download from the NIHR website, www.nihr.ac.uk.

Further reading

AFP

- General Medical Council's section on Ethical guidance for doctors – www.gmc-uk.org/ethical-guidance/ethical-guidance-for-doctors
  - *The Duties of a Doctor Registered with the General Medical Council* (available at: www.gmc-uk.org/ethical-guidance/ethical-guidance-for-doctors/good-medical-practice/duties-of-a-doctor)
  - *Good Medical Practice* (available at: www.gmc-uk.org/ethical-guidance/ethical-guidance-for-doctors/good-medical-practice)
- UKFPO Applicant Guidance – www.foundationprogramme.nhs.uk/content/resource-bank

ACF

- ACF interview scoring criteria (updated yearly on www.nihr.ac.uk)
- ACF Posts and Run Through Training – www.nihr.ac.uk/our-research-community/NIHR-academy/nihr-training-programmes/integrated-academic-training-programme/integrated-academic-training/academic-clinical-fellowships/acf-posts-and-run-through-training.htm
- ACF shortlisting criteria (updated yearly on www.nihr.ac.uk)
- NIHR Academic Clinical Fellowships – www.nihr.ac.uk/our-research-community/NIHR-academy/nihr-training-programmes/integrated-academic-training-programme/academic-clinical-fellowship-acf.htm
- NIHR Academic Clinical Fellowships (ACFs) Recruitment Information Pack (updated yearly on www.nihr.ac.uk)
- NIHR ACF Academic Person Specification (updated yearly on www.nihr.ac.uk)
- NIHR ACF FAQs (updated yearly on www.nihr.ac.uk)

AFP and ACF

- Oriel – www.oriel.nhs.uk
- Picard, O., Wood, D. and Yuen, S. (2013) *Medical Interviews: a comprehensive guide to CT, ST & Registrar interview skills*, 2nd edition. London: ISC Medical.

CHAPTER 4

The academic portfolio

Give me six hours to chop down a tree and I will
spend the first four sharpening the axe.

– ABRAHAM LINCOLN –

Throughout your career, you will often be asked at interview, for clinical and academic posts alike, to present a portfolio of achievement. Your portfolio is a record of your academic, clinical and extra-curricular attainment to date and it is something that you will carry with you throughout your career. The sooner you begin building it up, the stronger it will be.

The portfolio component of most interviews is given equal weighting to the other aspects, such as clinical, management, communication skills and practical procedures. However, it is the only part of the selection process where you can know roughly how well you have scored before you even set foot into the interview. You have full control over what goes into your portfolio and have the advantage of time to build and shape it towards the requirement of your desired specialty. Hence, it's worth reiterating that the sooner you start preparing this, the stronger a candidate you will be.

Hindsight is a wonderful thing; foresight would be even better but in the absence of the latter there is a lot of wisdom to be gained from the former. When beginning to compile evidence for your portfolio it is worth thinking about what the next 'bottleneck' in your training pathway is. As a medical student that bottleneck will likely be the FP or AFP application, whereas as a foundation trainee it will be specialty training or perhaps an ACF application. Once settled on a path, acquaint yourself with a person specification. For most training specialties, a link to the person specification can be found on the Health Education England Specialty training website (see the *Further reading* section at the end of the chapter).

Arguably as a medical student you should be looking beyond foundation training as all UK trainees are, barring any untoward events, guaranteed a foundation job. Therefore, the most advantageous measure to take at this stage will be to familiarise yourself with a specialty person specification (this includes core surgical training and core medical training). This will enable you to gear your portfolio towards addressing the required and desirable characteristics listed in the person specification. It will also focus your energy on tasks and pursuits that will yield points when it comes to specialty selection and not just add extra lines to your CV. Once you have identified areas of weakness in terms of your current ability to meet the person specification requirements, it would be useful at this stage to draw up a plan of action to address these deficiencies. Set realistic and achievable time-frames for addressing the areas in which you want to improve, and review your progress regularly. Be mindful that the person specification for specialty applications is updated yearly so be sure to keep up to date with any changes, should they occur.

4.1 What do I include in my portfolio?

Most clinically-based portfolios conform to a similar pattern in terms of included content and organisation. A typical structure is shown in *Box 4.1*.

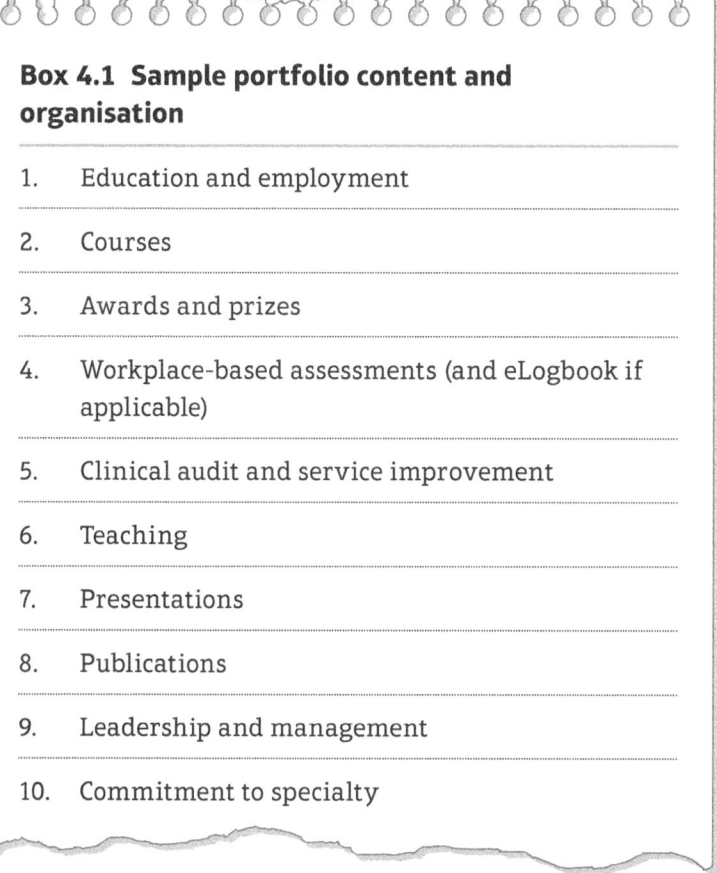

Box 4.1 Sample portfolio content and organisation

1. Education and employment

2. Courses

3. Awards and prizes

4. Workplace-based assessments (and eLogbook if applicable)

5. Clinical audit and service improvement

6. Teaching

7. Presentations

8. Publications

9. Leadership and management

10. Commitment to specialty

We will now explore each of the items in *Box 4.1* in terms of the practical evidence to include in your portfolio. Each section of your portfolio should start with a summary sheet serving as a mini-Contents page for the section.

1. Education and employment

This section should start with a CV that summarises everything in your portfolio and should roughly mirror the order and content of the portfolio. Following your CV you should include all undergraduate (including intercalated) and postgraduate degree certificates with evidence of level of award (1st, II:i, II:ii or 3rd class degree) or honours achieved (distinction or merit).

FAQ: Should I do an intercalated or additional degree including postgraduate certificates, diplomas or masters?

Additional degrees often score extra points during application, shortlisting and occasionally longlisting processes. They also give you lots of credit at fellowship applications later on in your training. However, the effort required to achieve these additional points, in the grand scheme of the selection process, is disproportionately great.

The bottom line is that if you have the chance to do an intercalated degree as part of your primary undergraduate degree, then go for it. This will often be funded, and most will provide you with early exposure to clinical or laboratory research. Furthermore, this will score you points on the application for the AFP and at core medical, surgical and specialty interviews. Any further additional degrees should be done on the basis of personal interest and motivation, not solely or primarily for the purpose of bolstering a portfolio.

You may also wish to include evidence of postgraduate certificates or diplomas, whether specifically relevant to your chosen specialty or not. Items of additional achievement may also be included, such as, for example, a Private Pilot's Licence or an Association Board of the Royal Schools of Music certificate. A general principle with your portfolio is to include as many items of evidence as possible. When approaching interview you can then trim off items that may be less applicable or those items not required.

It is also good practice to include a copy of your most recent General Medical Council (GMC) certificate of registration. Following this you may give a brief summation of your employment since graduation from your primary undergraduate degree.

FAQ: How much weight is placed on the level of award of additional degrees?

The selection committee is aware that not everyone will achieve a first-class degree; however, this is no excuse not to strive to attain one. The bottom line is that achieving a first-class degree will indeed make you positively stand out from the crowd and in some cases, will earn extra points during selection. However, this only forms one aspect of an extensive portfolio and selection process.

---

2. Courses

Throughout your career you will have to undertake courses to provide evidence of Continuing Professional Development (CPD). Some courses are specifically awarded CPD points, which as a medical student or trainee you are not required to collect. CPD points become important upon gaining your Certificate of Completion of Training. However, as with everything in the portfolio – the sooner you start, the better. A number of courses that are mandatory later on in your training can be done immediately or shortly after completing medical school. Furthermore, some courses specifically for medical students may attract points during selection for specialty training. For example, a colleague of mine attended a Royal College of Surgeons Summer School in Anatomy in the summer vacation following their second year of medical school, before they had settled on a career in surgery.

> **FAQ: Aside from the courses stated in person specifications, what other courses would you recommend attending?**
>
> In terms of non-mandatory courses, it is useful to be guided by your interests but be prepared to explain why you attended the course if asked to elaborate at interview. Generally speaking, it may be useful to attend a course on management and leadership and teaching skills in order to provide evidence of this. However, courses can be expensive to attend, especially if your study budgets do not cover the costs, so be judicious in your choices.

Six years later they found that attendance on that course attracted points on the core surgical training application.

The best place to look when thinking about what course to attend is the relevant person specification for the next stage of your training. These will often state the required or desirable courses. I would advocate attempting to attend all the courses stated by the time of application. If you are a medical student look at the courses required for core medical or surgical training or general practice (GP) training, whichever is applicable. Indeed, you may even want to look at the courses required for specialty applications.

> **FAQ: I have booked onto a course mentioned in the person specification, but it takes place after my interview. Should I include my booking confirmation?**
>
> Yes. Technically speaking, most interviewers should only give you a point for courses that you have completed and passed and for which you can provide evidence of attendance in the form of a certificate. However, some may recognise your intention to complete the course, and as the overwhelming majority of people pass the required courses, they may give you the credit. The bottom line is: if in doubt, include it.

3. Awards and prizes

In this section, you should include evidence of any distinctions or merits awarded during undergraduate and postgraduate training.

Prizes and awards can be for any aspect of your medical training to date and can even include those awarded from extra-curricular activities. It is good practice to provide a summary sheet listing the name of the award or prize, the awarding body, the date awarded and whether it was an undergraduate or postgraduate achievement or a national or international award.

Prizes and awards may vary from those awarded for excellent achievement during your degree, to those awarded for research projects, presentations or essay competitions. Research fellowships or bursaries may count for points in some specialty applications, because such awards involve a competitive selection process. If in doubt, include the evidence.

Unfortunately, a single compendium of medical prizes and awards doesn't exist, and some research is required to find them. However, prizes are frequently run by the Royal Society of Medicine, the British Medical Association and a number of Royal Colleges. It is also important to stress that failure is not absolute, and inability to win a prize at the first attempt should not mean you give up. A colleague of mine submitted their intercalated BSc project for a national prize and was disappointed to find that they had been unsuccessful and had not even been shortlisted. They continued to work on the project, however, were successful in getting it published in an international journal and re-submitted the project (largely unchanged) the following year. They won first place. Ultimately, you've got to be in it to win it! Many people are put off applying for prizes because they think they will never win. What they fail to understand is that everyone else is thinking exactly the same thing. However, the few who apply despite their inhibitions have greatly improved odds. I've heard of many stories of national prizes having only two applicants or submissions.

> **FAQ: How much weight is placed on merits and distinctions?**
>
> The selection committee is aware that not everyone will achieve a distinction or merit. These are often reserved for the top centiles of a year and thus the proportion achieving such may change each year. The bottom line is that achieving a distinction or merit will indeed make you positively stand out from the crowd and in some cases, will earn extra points during selection. However, as with additional degrees, this only forms one aspect of an extensive portfolio and selection process.

4. Workplace-based assessments

This section should include evidence of any clinical or procedural experience that you have attained, where acquisition of such is pertinent to your desired future career specialism. Such experience does not necessarily have to have been gained in the particular specialism in which you wish to practise. For instance, you may have had a chance to perform a percutaneous tracheostomy whilst on an ICU rotation. If you were able to complete a workplace-based assessment (WBA) for this procedure, it would be valuable evidence for a portfolio for an aspiring ENT trainee.

It is also useful to include evidence of multi-source feedback gained from your colleagues in the WBA section. This provides your interviewers with what is, hopefully, an accurate assessment of your character as a trainee and a far more comprehensive assessment than they are able to make within the time constraints of an interview.

Forms of evidence that you may wish to provide in the WBA section include:

✓ Letter from educational supervisor confirming experience

✓ Written evidence of completion of undergraduate specialist modules

✓ Evidence of reflection

✓ Evidence of internships confirming attainment of transferable skills

✓ Letters of commendation

✓ Patient feedback (including negative feedback, if you have reflected on it).

5. Clinical audit and service improvement

This section is self-explanatory, in that it provides a contemporaneous record of your involvement and commitment to quality improvement and audit. Ideally you should aim to lead and complete one closed audit cycle (including a re-audit), as this will earn you maximum points at interview. If you have presented your audit, whether regionally or further afield, or even been able to publish your audit, this is the section to scream and shout about it. The presentation itself may not necessarily score you additional points in this section but it does give the interviewers an appreciation of the scale and impact of your work and that it is more than just a tick-box activity for you. It is also worth bearing in mind that one completed 'closed loop' audit is worth significantly more than several audits that have been started but have not been seen through to completion. If time is a limiting factor it is better to put your efforts into completing one audit that can realistically be finished in a manageable timeframe than to be over-ambitious with several projects.

You should also include any evidence of ongoing participation in local audits or service improvement projects and ongoing re-audit projects. Increasingly with collaborative research networks it is becoming even easier to get involved with national audits, with almost minimal work needed compared to leading your own audit.

> **FAQ: Should I get involved with collaborative audits or just focus on leading and completing local audits?**
>
> Primarily your focus should be on completing as many meaningful audits as a lead as possible. However, there are benefits to collaborative audits in that they show evidence of teamwork within the collaborative research model. Most of these audits are national and thus have a wide-ranging impact, and are often presented and published in high impact factor journals. For the amount of effort required to participate in a collaborative audit, it provides a high yield of benefit. There are of course some disadvantages, in that it is very unlikely you will be involved in leading the entire audit, although you may be your local lead. Additionally, you may not be able to present it as you are not the lead and you may not be able to close the audit cycle. The bottom line is, you must prioritise leading and completing an audit. Beyond this, by all means participate in collaborative audits.

6. Teaching

This section provides an opportunity to describe and provide evidence of your teaching experience to date, whether that is informal, formal or near peer-led.

There are many different ways of getting involved in teaching. As a senior medical student, you may choose to set up a near peer-led teaching programme or participate in teaching that is run and delivered by your medical education society. You are uniquely placed, having only recently been in your junior colleagues' position; you may therefore be best positioned to deliver teaching in the most accessible and appropriate way. As a foundation doctor or trainee wanting to teach medical students, make contact with the local medical school affiliated with your hospital. Often student societies run teaching programmes throughout the year and advertise for trainees to deliver sessions. There is often a teaching need already identified and it is simply a matter of fulfilling a need. Where teaching needs have not been identified, it may be useful to survey students, enquiring about what they would like extra teaching or revision on and then creating a teaching programme, with the endorsement of the appropriate members of staff, that you can then deliver. Trainees and foundation doctors who have medical students rotate through their departments may want to enquire about additional teaching needs directly or approach the hospital medical education department. Most hospital education departments would be pleased to have additional help in delivering clinical skills teaching for medical students.

If you do establish a teaching programme, whether at your local hospital or university, make sure to issue certificates of attendance in exchange for feedback on the teaching. The feedback will prove extremely useful evidence in this section of your portfolio. If you are quite savvy you may wish to collect feedback before and after your teaching intervention to determine whether it has made a self-reported difference to your students or whether there has been an objective improvement in knowledge. Such assessments may form the basis of a small observational research project and some organisations, including the Association for the Study of Medical Education, welcome such projects at their annual conference.

Those who are passionate about teaching may consider taking a year out of formal training to do teaching fellow jobs which combine part-time clinical practice with a part-time teaching role. These roles often come with a funded postgraduate certificate or diploma in teaching which can be useful additional evidence in your portfolio. You do not have to do a teaching fellow job in order to undertake a formal teaching qualification, but outside of these roles you often have to self-fund the course and combine it with a full-time job. Such qualifications are not to be undertaken lightly as they are a significant burden in terms of time required to complete modules and assessments.

Forms of evidence that you may wish to provide in the teaching section include:

✓ Letter detailing your teaching achievement to date

✓ Certificate for attending a teaching course

✓ Letter confirming attainment of teaching skills

✓ Letter confirming involvement in a teaching programme

✓ Copy or copies of teaching completed (presentations delivered)

✓ Summary of teaching feedback received – best presented with a mixture of graphs and free text comments.

FAQ: I worked as a private tutor during medical school; should I include evidence of this in my portfolio?

My answer would be yes, even if you tutored in something non-medical, for example as a piano teacher. The fact that you show commitment to teaching matters more than the subject matter of the teaching.

FAQ: Do I need to collect feedback from all my teaching, even brief bedside teaching?

The point of this section is to show and document your ability to teach, and ultimately, having feedback from tutees shows this. Unless you have created formal lesson plans and accompanying presentations it is very hard to prove that you have delivered teaching. Having feedback forms from students, ideally with comments on what worked well and what could be improved, is undeniable evidence of your teaching.

7. Presentations

Evidence for this section encompasses all work presented at either a regional, national or international meeting. Often work that has only been presented locally will not score marks at interview. The presentations may have been by way of a poster or an oral presentation.

To build evidence for this section, the sooner you start, the better your portfolio will be. With any research project or audit that you undertake, no matter how small, you should always aim to achieve the 'golden trio' of a presentation (poster or oral), a prize (best poster / oral presentation or best research project) and a publication. In reality, it is very difficult to do this for every research project you do. However, the fact that it can be achieved highlights that doing a good research project can be potentially very high yielding if you do happen to achieve the golden trio, and will potentially score you maximum points in three out of the ten sections of your portfolio station.

Forms of evidence that you may wish to provide in the presentation section include:

✓ Copy of the presentation
  – poster: colour A4
  – oral: colour slides in handout view

✓ Copy of the event programme showing your name and the title of your presentation.

> **FAQ: I am the first author on a research project that my colleague presented – should I include this?**
>
> Although I would recommend you include this in your portfolio, you may not necessarily score points at interview for it. This is because you haven't actually delivered the presentation. However, including it in your portfolio does demonstrate the breadth of your research experience and previous work done.

FAQ: I am a collaborator (i.e. not first author) on a number of projects that have been presented by others – should I include these?

As with the previous question, I would encourage inclusion of these presentations. However, be mindful that some interview panels will only be interested in presentations that you have delivered, either as lead author or as a collaborator.

FAQ: I am not the first author on a project but I delivered the presentation at the conference – should I include this?

If you delivered the presentation then you should include this in your portfolio. Ensure that you are able to answer questions about the project and your role in the research, if asked at interview.

8. Publications

Depending on the job that you are applying for, this section will carry varying weight in terms of the points it will score you at interview. Obviously if you are applying for an academic post, you need to ensure that you come across strongly in terms of your research experience and output.

Ideally you should present the first page of each of your publications in this section. It is good practice to highlight your name in the author list, and this immediately indicates whether you are first author or not. If you have published a number of articles then perhaps choose only a selection of those in the highest impact factor journals, or those pertinent to the particular post that you are applying for. This section should primarily contain research that has been published in a recognised index such as Medline (PubMed). However, if you do not have many such indexed publications, do include those accepted elsewhere in non-indexed journals or non-peer-reviewed journals.

FAQ: I've published a few letters to the editor and case reports – should I include these?

The answer to this depends entirely on what else you have published. If you have published a number of high- or even medium-quality research projects, even if not in very high impact factor journals, then I would argue that the letters and case reports don't necessarily need to be included. Letters and case reports form the lowest level of evidence in terms of research and therefore you should consider including more items that are higher levels of evidence. That said, if you do not have any published research projects then definitely include these items.

It is worthwhile including letters of acceptance for research that has not yet been published. Again, identify the level of your authorship, and if it is not clear from the information in the letter, provide an abstract of the research to explain the nature of the project.

FAQ: Should I include published abstracts for presentations that I have delivered?

This is a common question that is asked. On the one hand, the presentation will form a part of your portfolio already in the previous presentation section. You may well have also published the full article in a high impact factor peer-reviewed journal. If you have met all the preceding criteria, then including a published abstract will add very little to your portfolio by way of prestige or points. I see published abstracts just as evidence of having presented your specified research at the specified conference that a journal supported, and nothing more. Some abstracts do end up being indexed in reputable archives. However, it does not take much digging to find that these are merely on abstracts and not complete research. The long and short of it is, include published abstracts as proof of conference attendance, but do not expect them to score you additional points in terms of additional publications.

9. Leadership and management

This section should be where you showcase your experience of having been in positions of leadership. Such positions can include roles held in medical school and indeed extra-curricular roles such as sports captaincy. Throughout your training, you need to show evidence of participating in teams, whether this is in the form of regional, national or international committees or otherwise.

There are many potential ways of getting involved with committees as a student or trainee, as many organisations have specific roles available for such members, including some Royal Colleges, trainee organisations and Royal Societies. This section would also be the place to include any roles that you have held on interview panels, in mentorship or in widening access initiatives. If you have a postgraduate qualification in management and/or leadership that has already been mentioned in Section 1 (*Education and employment*) you do not need to mention it again here. It may be useful, however, to include any projects undertaken as part of the work submitted towards the qualification.

Potential suitable roles during medical school:

- Society committee member or chair
- University sports teams.

Potential suitable roles as a trainee:

- Trainee representative
- Role within the doctors' mess
- Departmental responsibilities (e.g. rota coordinator).

Forms of evidence that you may wish to provide in the *Leadership and management* section include:

✓ Original letter from medical school / departments / foundation school / national or international organisation

✓ Original certificate

✓ Letter of appreciation.

10. Commitment to specialty

This section really allows you to show the lengths to which you have gone to improve your experience of, and awareness about your desired specialty. It is a great opportunity to include evidence that may not quite be suitable for other sections of your portfolio, but which nonetheless strengthens it.

Forms of evidence that you may wish to provide in the *Commitment to specialty* section include:

✓ Specific specialty-level skills, e.g. practical procedures

✓ Specific experience or training (e.g. posts, specialist clinics, etc.)

✓ Specialty-related research or grants applied for that have not yet resulted in a presentation or publication

✓ Membership of relevant societies, committees or organisations

✓ Specialty-themed elective

✓ Certificates showing success at relevant specialty exams

✓ Certificates of attendance at relevant conferences

✓ Evidence of a taster week, or shadowing, with a written reflective account of the experience.

Further reading

- The Association for the Study of Medical Education (ASME) – www.asme.org.uk/
- Health Education England: Person specification – https://specialtytraining.hee.nhs.uk/Recruitment/Person-specifications

CHAPTER 5

Introduction to epidemiology for interviews

Far better an approximate answer to the right question, which is often vague, than an exact answer to the wrong question, which can always be made precise.

– JOHN W. TUKEY –

If you are reading this book it is likely that you will have some background knowledge of epidemiology and at least basic skills in critical appraisal. As you will see in this chapter, many academic interviews have a component of critical appraisal, or at least a discussion surrounding academic methods. As such, it is imperative that you thoroughly equip yourself beforehand in order to tackle any questions that may be directed your way. Karl Pearson, the esteemed mathematician, once remarked that, "Statistics is the grammar of science." Indeed, familiarising yourself with basic principles of statistics and epidemiology will serve you well in furnishing your answers to the research questions directed at you.

5.1   Courses and academic skills

If you are successful in being appointed to an academic training programme, your training will involve undertaking more advanced courses in research methods and governance. However, in keeping with the running theme of this book, early preparation will set you apart. This will particularly be the case if you are already familiar with these courses and research interviews by the time of your interview.

Good clinical practice

"Good clinical practice is a set of internationally recognised ethical and scientific quality requirements which must be observed for designing, conducting, recording and reporting clinical trials that involve the participation of human subjects. Compliance with this good practice provides assurance that the rights, safety and well-being of trial subjects are protected, and that the results of the clinical trials are credible" states the European Commission's Clinical Trials Directive 2001/20/EC. In the UK, the majority of research ethics committees will require proof of good clinical practice (GCP) compliance if you are a principal applicant for ethics approval on research using human tissue or will be working in a lab conducting such research. Most universities will offer a GCP course for researchers within their departments but there are an increasing number of national courses, not affiliated to a university, that you may wish to attend prior to your interview. Attendance at a GCP course is by no means necessary prior to applying for an academic job. However, familiarisation with the principles of GCP is highly recommended.

Research governance

GCP and research governance overlap; familiarising yourself with GCP will improve your understanding of research governance which is a topic that is frequently asked about at interviews, but is often poorly answered. As with GCP courses, research governance courses are available through universities and also external organisations. These courses explore the Department of Health research governance framework, known as the UK Policy Framework for Health and Social Care Research. This framework covers core standards that govern numerous domains within research, including ethics, regulatory bodies, participant health and safety, transparency and intellectual property. For more information on GCP and the Department of Health research governance framework, see the *Further reading* section at the end of this chapter.

Statistical methods

Whilst it is useful to attend a course on statistical methods in preparation for your academic interview, this is not compulsory. However, as with the GCP and research governance courses, you may find your experience on them beneficial, as they will explore medical statistics and epidemiological methods in greater detail than the scope of this book allows. Alternatively you could consider reading a good introductory text to medical statistics; a number of good books are mentioned in the *Further reading* section at the end of this chapter.

5.2   Defining a research question

A research question can be broken down into the following four factors; the acronym PICO serves as a useful reminder of these factors and is also a useful basis to begin a critical appraisal of any paper reporting a primary study.

P   The **p**opulation of interest

I   The treatment or healthcare **i**ntervention to be investigated

C   The **c**omparator or **c**ontrol group to which the treatment group receiving the intervention will be compared

O   **O**utcome measure(s) of the intervention.

5.3 Describing diagnostic tests

Sensitivity and specificity are the key parameters for describing diagnostic tests:

- **Sensitivity**: the probability that a person with a condition of interest will test positive
- **Specificity**: the probability that a person without a condition of interest will test negative.

These can be calculated using *Table 5.1.*

Table 5.1 Two-way table

Test result	Condition present	Condition absent
Positive	A (true positive)	B (false positive)
Negative	C (false negative)	D (true negative)

Sensitivity: $\dfrac{A}{(A+C)}$ OR $\dfrac{\text{true positive}}{(\text{true positive} + \text{false negative})}$

Specificity: $\dfrac{D}{(D+B)}$ OR $\dfrac{\text{true negative}}{(\text{true negative} + \text{false positive})}$

Table 5.1 can also be used to describe **positive and negative predictive value**:

- **Positive predictive value**: the probability that a person with a positive result has the condition of interest
- **Negative predictive value**: the probability that a person with a negative result does not have the condition of interest.

Positive predictive value: $\dfrac{A}{(A+B)}$

Negative predictive value: $\dfrac{D}{(D+C)}$

5.4 Reporting guidelines

Historically, healthcare research reporting was non-standardised, with varying degrees of reporting quality. Common problems in research reporting included failure to report on an intention-to-treat analysis basis, use of surrogate or composite outcomes, multiple subgroup analyses, presentation of relative rather than absolute benefits, and omission of reporting on adverse effects.

In order to improve the reporting of clinical research, various guidelines have been developed. Many journals now insist that authors wanting to publish in their journals conform to the relevant reporting guideline for their respective article. Frequently employed reporting guidelines are shown in *Table 5.2*.

Table 5.2 Reporting guidelines used in healthcare research

Study type	Reporting guideline
Randomised trials	CONSORT
Observational studies	STROBE
Systematic reviews	PRISMA
Study protocols	PRISMA-P, SPIRIT
Diagnostic/prognostic studies	STARD, TRIPOD
Case reports	CARE
Clinical practice guidelines	AGREE, RIGHT
Qualitative research	SRQR, COREQ
Animal pre-clinical studies	ARRIVE
Quality improvement studies	SQUIRE
Economic evaluations	CHEERS

For more information on these guidelines see under the relevant heading in the *Further reading* section at the end of this chapter.

5.5 Patient Reported Outcome Measures

Patient Reported Outcome Measures (PROMs) are self-reported perspectives of health, functional status and quality of life (QoL), which often measure the effect of different healthcare interventions on disease state. They are typically assessed through standardised and validated questionnaires.

The concept of PROMs originated in clinical trials where they assessed the effectiveness of different healthcare interventions. They are now becoming increasingly common within clinical practice where they help to inform patient management on a patient-specific basis. First introduced into clinical practice in the UK in 2008 in an audit of mastectomy and breast reconstruction, PROMs were then introduced into routine practice in assessing patient outcomes in elective hip and knee replacement, groin hernia repair and varicose vein surgery. Since 2013 PROMs have been included in the NHS Outcome Framework.

Uses of PROMs:

- Clinical trials – PROMs data can provide evidence on treatment effectiveness within large cohorts
- Monitoring disease progression
- Stimulating improvements in the quality of healthcare delivery, by acting as a means to compare healthcare provider outcomes
- National audits and registers
- Screening tools
- Identifying patient preferences and guiding decision making with regard to treatment
- Improving patient–provider communication.

PROMs can be largely divided into two categories: generic and disease-specific. Generic PROMs focus on a global assessment of health-related quality of life, whereas disease-specific PROMs assess quality of life in light of a patient's particular disease burden or morbidity. *Table 5.3* gives examples of some PROMs currently in use.

Table 5.3 Examples of PROMs

PROM	Disease focus	User	Items	Scoring
Euro – Quality of Life Question-naire (EQ-5D)	Generic	Patient-completed	6	3 or 5 level scale
Short Form Survey 36 (SF-36)	Generic	Patient-completed	36	2–6 response options
University of Washington Quality of Life Questionnaire (UW-QoL)	Generic	Patient-completed	12	3–6 response options
Sino-Nasal Outcome Test 20	Disease-specific – ENT	Patient-completed	20	6-point Likert scale

Further reading

- The Equator Network – www.equator-network.org/
- Good Clinical Practice – European Commission directive 2001/20/EC
- Greenhalgh, T. (2014) *How to Read a Paper: the basics of evidence-based medicine*, 5th edition. Oxford: Wiley-Blackwell.
- Harris, G. and Taylor, G. (2014) *Medical Statistics Made Easy*, 3rd edition. Banbury: Scion Publishing.
- NHS Health Research Authority (2018) *UK Policy Framework for Health and Social Care Research*. Available at: www.hra.nhs.uk/planning-and-improving-research/policies-standards-legislation/uk-policy-framework-health-social-care-research/
- Peacock, J. and Peacock, P. (2010) *Oxford Handbook of Medical Statistics*. Oxford: Oxford University Press.
- Ward, H., Toledano, M.B., Shaddick, G. *et al.* (2012) *Oxford Handbook of Epidemiology for Clinicians*. Oxford: Oxford University Press.

AGREE

- Brouwers, M.C., Kerkvliet, K. and Spithoff, K.; AGREE Next Steps Consortium (2016) The AGREE Reporting Checklist: a tool to improve reporting of clinical practice guidelines. *BMJ*, **352:**i1152.

ARRIVE

- Kilkenny, C., Browne, W.J., Cuthill, I.C. *et al.* (2010) Improving bioscience research reporting: the ARRIVE guidelines for reporting animal research. *PLoS Biology*, **8(6):** e1000412.

CARE

- Gagnier, J.J., Kienle, G., Altman, D.G. *et al.*; the CARE Group (2013) The CARE Guidelines: consensus-based clinical case reporting guideline development. *BMJ Case Reports*, doi: 10.1136/bcr-2013-201554.

CHEERS

- Husereau, D., Drummond, M., Petrou, S. *et al.* (2013) Consolidated Health Economic Evaluation Reporting Standards (CHEERS) statement. *European Journal of Health Economics*, **14(3):** 367–372.

CONSORT

- Schulz, K.F., Altman, D.G. and Moher, D.; for the CONSORT Group (2010) CONSORT 2010 Statement: updated guidelines for reporting parallel group randomized trials. *Annals of Internal Medicine*, **152(11):** 726–732.

COREQ

- Tong, A., Sainsbury, P. and Craig, J. (2007) Consolidated criteria for reporting qualitative research (COREQ): a 32-item checklist for interviews and focus groups. *International Journal for Quality in Health Care*, **19(6):** 349–357.

PRISMA

- Moher, D., Liberati, A., Tetzlaff, J. *et al.* (2009) Preferred Reporting Items for Systematic Reviews and Meta-Analyses: the PRISMA statement. *Annals of Internal Medicine*, **151(4):** 264–269.

PRISMA-P

- Moher, D., Shamseer, L., Clarke, M. *et al.* (2015) Preferred Reporting Items for Systematic Review and Meta-Analysis Protocols (PRISMA-P) 2015 statement. *Systematic Reviews*, **4(1):** 1.

RIGHT

- Chen, Y., Yang, K., Marušić, A. *et al.*; for the RIGHT (Reporting Items for Practice Guidelines in Healthcare) Working Group (2017) A reporting tool for practice guidelines in health care: the RIGHT statement. *Annals of Internal Medicine*, **166(2):** 128–132.

SPIRIT

- Chan, A-W., Tetzlaff, J.M., Altman, D.G. *et al.* (2013) SPIRIT 2013 Statement: defining standard protocol items for clinical trials. *Annals of Internal Medicine*, **158(3):** 200–207.

SQUIRE

- Ogrinc, G., Davies, L., Goodman, D. *et al.* (2016) SQUIRE 2.0 (*Standards for QUality Improvement Reporting Excellence*): revised publication guidelines from a detailed consensus process. *BMJ Quality & Safety*, **25:** 986–992.

SRQR

- O'Brien, B.C., Harris, I.B., Beckman, T.J. *et al.* (2014) Standards for reporting qualitative research: a synthesis of recommendations. *Academic Medicine*, **89(9):** 1245–1251.

STARD

- Bossuyt, P.M., Reitsma, J.B., Bruns, D.E. *et al.*; for the STARD Group (2015) STARD 2015: an updated list of essential items for reporting diagnostic accuracy studies. *BMJ*, **351:**h5527.

STROBE

- von Elm, E., Altman, D.G., Egger, M. *et al.* (2007) The Strengthening the Reporting of Observational Studies in Epidemiology (STROBE) Statement: guidelines for reporting observational studies. *Annals of Internal Medicine*, **147(8):** 573–577.

TRIPOD

- Collins, G.S., Reitsma, J.B., Altman, D.G. and Moons, K.G. (2015) Transparent Reporting of a multivariable prediction model for Individual Prognosis Or Diagnosis (TRIPOD): the TRIPOD statement. *Annals of Internal Medicine*, **162(1):** 55–63.

CHAPTER 6

The interview

*You don't practise 'til you get it right, you
practise 'til you can't get it wrong.*

– OLIVE LEWIN –

The preparation needed to succeed at interview begins long before the interview takes place. By the time you have been offered your interview, you will have spent much time laying the foundations in place to be appointed to your academic post. The effort spent attending conferences, presenting research and writing and publishing papers is not in vain. In fact, as I have said previously, looking at someone's portfolio often gives you an idea of the person behind that portfolio and, bar a catastrophe on the day of the interview, the better portfolios often tend to accompany the successful candidates.

It is impossible to compile an exhaustive list of every possible question or topic that you may be asked about on the day of your interview, but nonetheless there is much that you can do to be better equipped than someone who goes in with no or little preparation.

6.1   Format of the interview

The format of your interview will vary from region to region and there is no set template. Most academic jobs, being linked to a clinical post, will require you to be successful in both the academic interview and a separate clinical interview. The AFP jobs have only one interview in which both your academic and clinical potential are assessed, as well as your suitability for the job applied for.

Academic interviews are typically split into a clinical assessment, an academic assessment and an assessment of your portfolio. Some interviews will specifically ask you to list evidence of certain academic achievements (e.g. first author publications and prizes, evidence of leadership or management) before the interview, while others may require you to bring certain items from your portfolio or your entire portfolio to the interview.

Before the interview, you may be given an abstract to critically appraise. In the case of AFP interviews, you may be given a handover sheet to triage, and subsequently be asked questions about clinical prioritisation. The academic interview may also cover questions about your teaching experience to date and plans for potential projects that you may wish to undertake during your academic rotation. Below are examples of the format of previous AFP and ACF interviews from successful candidates.

In order to improve your chances of success at interview it is worth practising what answers you will give to different interview questions. If at all possible, apply the idea of the pyramid of feedback discussed in *Chapter 3* in order to get comments on your question responses from various colleagues and thus refine your answers.

Format of previous AFP interviews

London (Imperial, UCL, King's, St George's, QMUL)

Clinical interview involving prioritisation and subsequent systematic assessment and initiation of initial management plan for acutely unwell patients. Academic interview based on the critical appraisal of an abstract provided twenty minutes prior to the interview.

Manchester

Clinical station starting with the review of several patient blood results followed by a discussion around the management of a number of medical and surgical scenarios. Further clinical scenario involved the discussion around GMC principles of Good Medical Practice and how these related to the specific scenarios.

Oxford

Clinical station involving the reading of multiple clinical vignettes and discussion of evidence-based patient management for each scenario. Academic station involving the discussion of academic achievements to date (publications, presentations and prizes), proposed plans for research during the AFP and in-depth discussion of a publication mentioned on submitted application.

Format of previous ACF interviews

London (UCL)

Three-person panel plus a lay person representative. Questions were asked about previous research experience to date – publications and projects. Discussion and questions around two clinical scenarios including assessment and initial management. No formal split between academic and clinical components of the interview.

Birmingham

Single interview, split into two sections. Candidate was initially asked about academic achievements to date, making reference to publications, prizes and awards mentioned on application. Discussion centred on explaining research projects and role in the projects. Subsequent discussion about the management of a basic clinical scenario related to the specialty of the ACF, including initial assessment and management and suggestions on managing potential complications.

6.2 Managing clinical emergencies

Everyone takes a different approach in terms of the way they tackle the management of an acutely unwell patient or a clinical scenario. There isn't necessarily a best way, you just need to make sure you cover the absolute basics, don't jeopardise patient safety and escalate appropriately and in a timely manner. *Box 6.1* shows a potential structure for managing any clinical scenario; note that it is not the only possible approach.

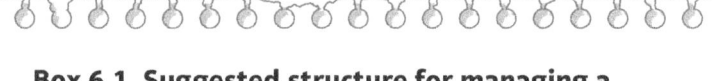

Box 6.1 Suggested structure for managing a clinical scenario

1. Opening gambit, e.g. "My immediate concern is ..."

2. Phone advice (if called in A&E to see someone on the ward)
   - ask the person on the phone to prepare op notes (if applicable), obs chart, fluid balance and other records for you

3. Emergency vs. elective

4. Focused history (AMPLE)

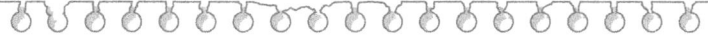

5. Examination
- ABCDE assessment including bedside investigations (VBG, lactate, glucose, FBC, U&Es)

6. Differential diagnosis and working diagnoses

7. Investigations and imaging

8. Initial plan of action
- including reassessment of patient status after each intervention

9. Management plan (stable patient vs. unstable patient)
- only state that you would perform tasks in which you are proficient – if, for example, a chest drain is needed and you'd never performed one, state, "I would ask for someone more proficient in insertion to perform the task"
- may involve escalation to senior colleague or at least making them and other specialties aware that input may be required from them (e.g. ICU, critical care outreach)

10. Important others: analgesia, pregnancy test in females, tetanus for open wounds

11. Governance (morbidity and mortality – M&M)
- does the relevant patient need to be recorded in the departmental M&M log?

12. Reflection

13. eLogbook/electronic portfolio (if applicable).

The structure shown in *Box 6.1* comprehensively covers a potential approach for tackling any clinical scenario in an interview environment. Whilst not all of the points listed may be applicable to every scenario you are given, it nevertheless forms a template that can be adapted as needed. Points 12 and 13 in *Box 6.1* don't deal with the management of the patient, but show that you are using the case to inform your ongoing learning.

CHAPTER 7

What to do if it doesn't go right first time

Success is not measured by the heights one attains, but by the obstacles one overcomes in its attainment.

– BOOKER T. WASHINGTON –

The road to academic success is not an easy one, otherwise there would be no shortage of clinical academics. Sometimes things don't always go to plan and despite the best intentions and preparation something untoward happens on the day of interview, or for whatever reason you are not successful in acquiring your dream job. It is inevitable to be frustrated with this outcome; however, don't let it dissuade you, cloud your judgement or dampen your self-belief. Learn from your mistakes and the mistakes and successes of others, as you'll never live long enough to make them all yourself.

If you were unsuccessful at the final hurdle I would encourage you to ask for feedback from the interview panel about your performance. You may well know where you fell short or it may surprise you. Even for those candidates who are reading this before the interview and go on to be appointed, it is useful to request feedback on your performance. You can always improve. If you are unsuccessful at interview, use the feedback received to formulate goals and achievable targets, whether this means acquiring additional evidence for your portfolio or better managing clinical scenarios. It is often invaluable to practise with peers as they may highlight blind spots in terms of your knowledge. In your preparation for re-application you may find it useful to write down where you want to be in, for example, five years' time. Reminding yourself of the end goal, and that this lies beyond the next interview, is an excellent motivator and focuses your mind and efforts. It's important to build a routine and form a habit around practice, whether this involves going through potential interview questions for an hour every evening or spending 30 minutes critically appraising a paper each morning on the way to work. The best preparation is the sort that you can build into your daily routine as it, in time, becomes incorporated into your natural activity. With the end goal in mind, it is useful to push yourself incrementally, in terms both of the type of material you challenge yourself with and the volume. Although time constraints may limit the volume with which you can challenge yourself, remember that your goal should be to see tangible progress so that the next time you come to the application and interview process, you won't need to read this chapter again!

INDEX

Related titles

Remember, you can order any Scion books at 35% discount from:
www.scionpublishing.com/medicalstudents

Simply add the books to your basket and enter the promotional code
scionpub35 when prompted.

*Whilst there, don't forget to sign up for our medical student newsletter to hear
first about new books, special offers, giveaways, etc.*

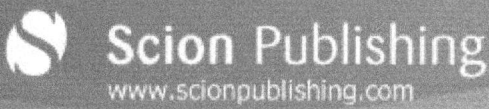

Welcome to the latest medical student newsletter
Scroll down for free samples.....

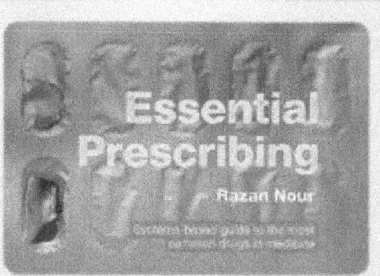

Just Published!

Essential Prescribing
Razan Nour
Apr 2018
Spiral bound - ISBN 9781911510000
Price: £19.99

View sample chapter here

Free Samples this month

Click to access free sample chapters

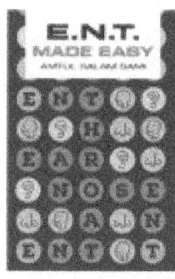
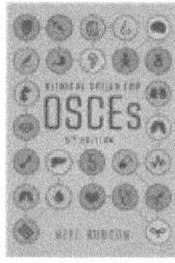
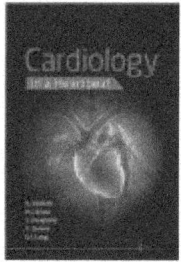
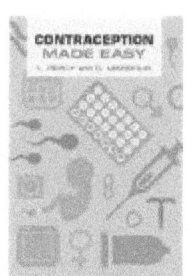

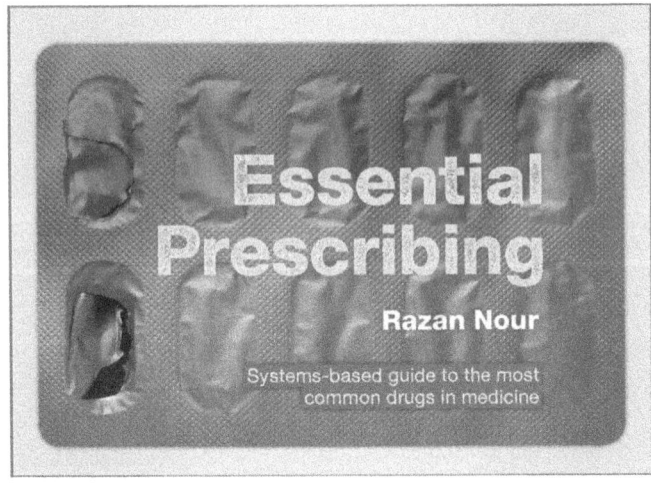

Essential Prescribing

Razan Nour

Spiral bound, 186pp, ISBN 9781911510000, Price: £19.99

Essential Prescribing is a brand new text aimed at providing medical students with an easy-to-follow overview of the drugs they are most likely to encounter at medical school and as they start their medical careers. The book benefits from the same landscape format and approach as Scion's bestselling *Essential Examination*.

Each class of drug is detailed using a common tabular format, based on the following sections:

Examples, Mode of Action, Routes of Delivery, Indications, Cautions and contraindications, Interactions, Monitoring, Side-effects, Patient counselling.

This consistent approach helps the reader quickly find the pertinent information for the common drugs and situations they are likely to come across, so they can become confident of prescribing the correct drugs for the patient in appropriate doses.

Review:

'This book is a wealth of information! Well written in a simple concise way, easy to follow guidelines for prescribing medications, oxygen, intravenous fluids ... and is divided by the system involved and has a section specifically for patient counselling which makes this book unique.' ★★★★★

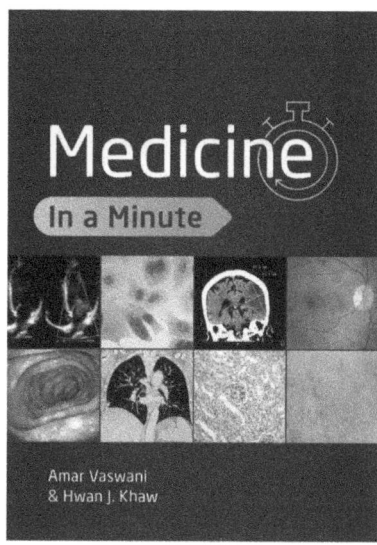

Medicine in a Minute

Amar Vaswani and Hwan Juet Khaw

Paperback, 504pp, ISBN 9781907904981, £29.99

Medicine in a Minute is a brand new full-colour text covering the fundamentals of undergraduate medicine in one book. Medical students no longer have the time or inclination to read the huge texts that used to dominate this market - they need a concise book that covers the core information they have to know, and in a user-friendly format: *Medicine in a Minute* is this book.

The book is edited and written by two of the authors behind the bestselling *Cardiology in a Heartbea*t and features several common design elements and features.

The book is divided into body systems and then each section within the particular body system follows a consistent pattern:

- Definition
- Differential diagnosis
- Clinical features
- Epidemiology
- Aetiology
- Investigations
- Risk factors
- Pathophysiology
- Management

Medicine in a Minute is a student-friendly, concise text that you will want close to hand throughout your studies.

Review:

'I've bought many medical textbooks during my time in medical school but I can simply say this is the best of its type. Pitched at exactly the right level for clinical medicine.'
★★★★★

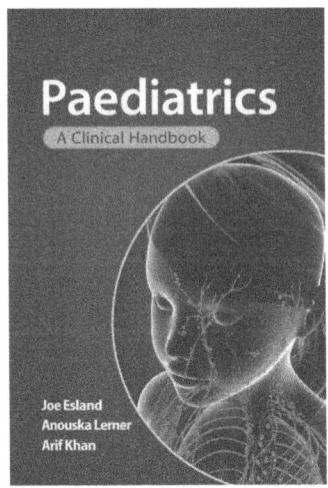

Paediatrics: A Clinical Handbook

Joe Esland, Anouska Lerner and Arif Khan

Paperback, 320pp, ISBN 9781907904851, Price: £23.99

Paediatrics: A Clinical Handbook provides all the essential information required for a successful paediatrics rotation. Written by two recently qualified junior doctors and a consultant paediatrician, the book offers an exam-centred, reader-friendly style backed up with concise clinical guidance.

Building on the success of the other 'Clinical Handbook' titles (*Rheumatology* and *Psychiatry*), *Paediatrics: A Clinical Handbook* provides student-friendly coverage of the material with many key features (such as mnemonics and OSCE tips) to help the reader get to grips with the subject.

Paediatrics: A Clinical Handbook is ideal for medical students and junior doctors; like the other books in the series it will have a secondary market amongst medics who want a quick refresher of the subject.

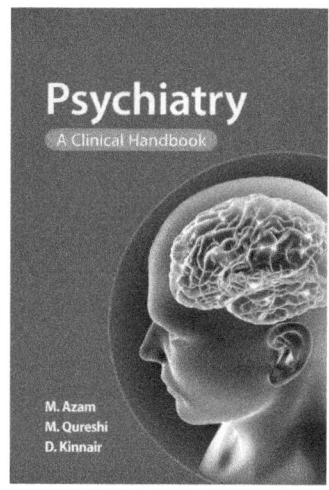

Use your QR reader
to access more
information and
sample material.

Psychiatry: A Clinical Handbook

Mohsin Azam, Mohammed Qureshi and Daniel Kinnair

Paperback, 282pp, ISBN 9781907904813, Price: £23.99

Psychiatry: A Clinical Handbook provides all the essential information required for a successful psychiatry rotation. Written by two recently qualified junior doctors and a consultant psychiatrist, the book offers an exam-centred, reader-friendly style backed up with concise clinical guidance.

The book covers diagnosis and management based upon the ICD-10 Classification and the latest NICE guidelines. For every psychiatric condition:

- the diagnostic pathway is provided with suggested phrasing for sensitive questions
- the relevant clinical features to look out for in the mental state examination are listed
- a concise definition and basic pathophysiology/aetiology is outlined.

Self-assessment questions are provided at the end of each chapter. A chapter is dedicated to OSCE scenarios to aid practising with colleagues in preparation for exams. SBA questions with detailed answers written by a Consultant Psychiatrist are also provided.

Reviews:

'One of the best psychiatry books I have ever read. It is organised in a neat, concise manner with tables, colours, mnemonics, OSCE tips to name but a few.' ★★★★★

'Great book for undergraduate psychiatry. Lots of useful mnemonics and colour coded to aid commit facts to memory.' ★★★★★

'Finally a psychiatry book great for quick referencing, with a design made for the modern reader.' ★★★★★

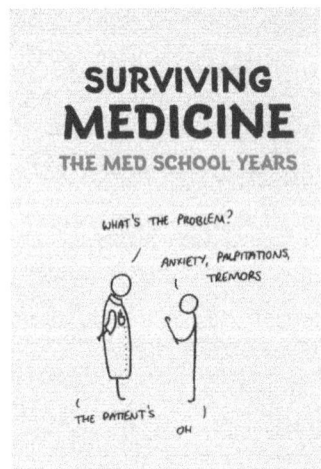

Surviving Medicine

Will Sloper

Paperback, 154pp, ISBN 9781911510253, Price: £14.99

Medicine is one of the most wonderfully ridiculous professions in the world and the cartoons in this book are light-hearted reflections on life as a medical student.

Most of the situations described in this book will crop up at some point as you progress through medical school and beyond. Consider them a rite of passage as you rack up the experience and confidence to look back and think, *I can't believe I was scared of that...!*

But more than that, the book offers advice on surviving ward rounds, coping with doubt and anxiety, preparing for exams, and lots more besides!

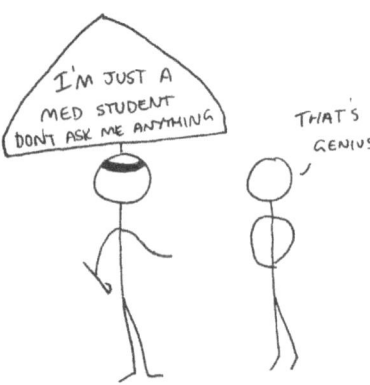